YOUR KNOWLEDGE HAS VALUE

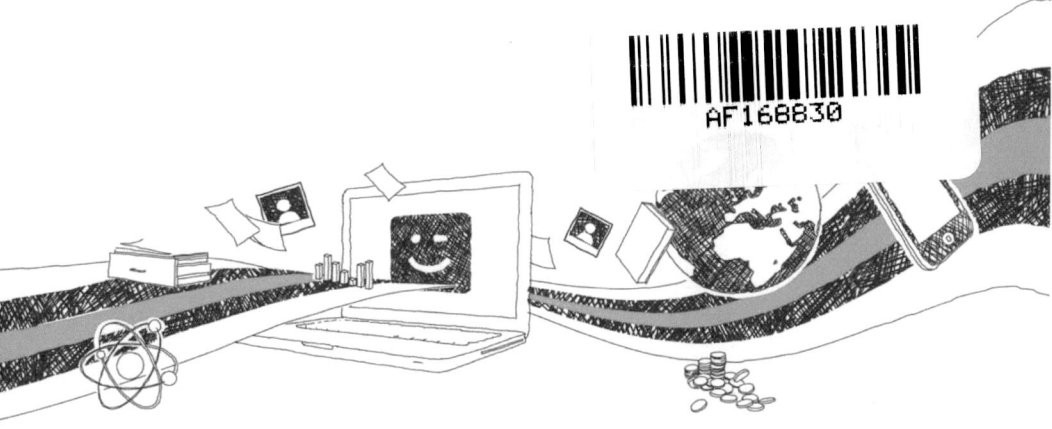

- We will publish your bachelor's and master's thesis, essays and papers

- Your own eBook and book - sold worldwide in all relevant shops

- Earn money with each sale

Upload your text at www.GRIN.com and publish for free

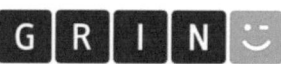

Bibliographic information published by the German National Library:

The German National Library lists this publication in the National Bibliography; detailed bibliographic data are available on the Internet at http://dnb.dnb.de .

This book is copyright material and must not be copied, reproduced, transferred, distributed, leased, licensed or publicly performed or used in any way except as specifically permitted in writing by the publishers, as allowed under the terms and conditions under which it was purchased or as strictly permitted by applicable copyright law. Any unauthorized distribution or use of this text may be a direct infringement of the author s and publisher s rights and those responsible may be liable in law accordingly.

Imprint:

Copyright © 2018 GRIN Verlag
Print and binding: Books on Demand GmbH, Norderstedt Germany
ISBN: 9783668741775

This book at GRIN:

https://www.grin.com/document/431376

Patrick Kimuyu

The Future of Nursing as Envisaged by the Institute of Medicine

GRIN Verlag

GRIN - Your knowledge has value

Since its foundation in 1998, GRIN has specialized in publishing academic texts by students, college teachers and other academics as e-book and printed book. The website www.grin.com is an ideal platform for presenting term papers, final papers, scientific essays, dissertations and specialist books.

Visit us on the internet:

http://www.grin.com/

http://www.facebook.com/grincom

http://www.twitter.com/grin_com

The Future of Nursing as Envisaged by the Institute of Medicine

Name: Patrick Kimuyu

Contents

Introduction 3

Key Messages 3

    Key Message #1 4

    Key Message #2 4

    Key Message #3 5

    Key Message #4 5

Recommendations 5

    Recommendation #1 6

    Recommendation #2 6

    Recommendation #3 7

    Recommendation #4 7

    Recommendation #5 8

    Recommendation #6 8

    Recommendation #7 9

    Recommendation #8 9

Conclusion 9

References 11

Introduction

In the recent years, nursing education and practice appear to have been influenced by the current healthcare reforms. The Affordable Care Act has introduced cross-sectional changes in the US healthcare system. For instance, it has led to an increase in the number of uninsured people by introducing universal healthcare under the reviewed health insurance plans. It is predicted that "expanding the reach of insurance coverage will place greater demands on the primary care system, as witnessed in Massachusetts" (IOM, 2010a p. 375). Consequently, the scope of healthcare services has experienced immense changes ranging from patient's privacy protection as it is defined by HIPAA to the treatment of degenerative diseases. IOM observes "primary care medical homes and accountable care organizations (ACOs)—rely on interventions that fall squarely within the scope of practice of RNs (e.g., care coordination, transitional care)" (p.375). Owing to these changes in the US healthcare system, transient reforms in the nursing profession are deemed necessary for addressing the vast needs of the US population, and this explains the importance of the 2010 Institute of Medicine's recommendations. Evidence indicates that, the nursing profession plays the pivotal role in the healthcare system because it accounts for the largest percentage of the healthcare workforce. As such, introducing transformations in the nursing profession appear to be as significant as the Affordable Care Act, especially regarding the improvement of healthcare service delivery. Therefore, this research paper will provide a comprehensive overview on the impact of IOM recommendations on the nursing profession including the key messages.

Key Messages

It is apparent that, the IOM report encompasses an array of aspects related to the nursing profession. These aspects seem to have a direct contribution to the recent reforms in the US healthcare reforms that are intended for promoting access to high quality healthcare services. Despite the fact that, some of the elements of healthcare reforms are meant to address the issue of increased healthcare costs in the US healthcare system, there are some elements that aim at improving service provision. As such, transforming the nursing profession appears to play a pivotal role in aligning the Affordable Care Act requirements in the US healthcare system. This is why IOM highlighted on four significant messages.

Key Message #1

The first key message is that, transforming the nursing practice requires nurses to employ their professional potential in the service delivery, in the healthcare system. This will be done through ensuring that nurses use their educational and training experience to the full extent. IOM (2010a) states "federal and state actions are required to update and standardize scope-of-practice regulations to take advantage of the full capacity and education of APRNs" (p. 29). This approach will ensure that, the nurses' contribution to the transformation of the US healthcare are maximized leading to enhanced access to quality healthcare services by all the American citizens. In accomplishing these requirements, it is suggested that states and insurance companies are supposed to carry out transient changes in their regulatory, policy and financial frameworks. In addition, it is reported that the nature of care in the US is likely going to experience a significant shift from the hospital to community settings. As such, transformation in the nursing practice needs to be done, in order to align it with the future changes. It is observed that, nurses are still confined in the acute care setting that is expected to change in the foreseeable future (IOM, 2010a).

Key Message #2

The second message in the IOM report is that, nurses should "achieve higher levels of education and training through an improved education system that promotes seamless academic progression" (p. 30). IOM observes that, changing the US healthcare system will require transient changes in the nursing education. It is believed that, nursing education plays a significant role in determining the quality of services provided by nurses in the care settings. Therefore, it is apparent that any significant change in the nursing education will lead to remarkable changes in the entire healthcare system. This is why IOM states "An improved education system is necessary to ensure that the current and future generations of nurses can deliver safe, quality, patient-centered care across all settings, especially in such areas as primary care and community and public health" (p. 30). However, it is worth noting that the nursing education covers both the period before and after the accreditation of nurses, primarily regarding their certification with nursing licenses.

It is interesting to note that; enrollment of students into the nursing profession has increased significantly in the past few decades. This implies that, the nursing workforce is going to expand in the future, and this will enhance service provision in the US healthcare system because the nurse-patient ratio will improve although there are some limitations.

Key Message #3

Key message 3 deals with the transformation of the nursing leadership to ensure that the administration of nursing is based on the most appropriate professional approaches. IOM observes that most nurses do not aspire to become leaders as part of their nursing profession, yet the intended transformation of the US healthcare system will require extensive nursing leadership. As such, nurses in the current and future care settings are expected to play the dual roles of offering services to patients and serving as stewards in the healthcare system by demonstrating sound leadership. This is why IOM (2010a) suggests "a transformed system will need nurses with the adaptive capacity to take on reconceptualized roles in new settings, educating and reeducating themselves along the way—indispensable characteristics of effective leadership" (p. 32). Consequently, nurses are advised to focus on policy as something that they can shape, but not necessarily something that they experience. In general, IOM reinstates the need for transforming the nursing leadership.

Key Message #4

On the other hand, IOM report that an improved information infrastructure that encompasses improved data collection will enhance workforce planning for efficient transformation of the entire healthcare system. Ordinarily, the US healthcare system comprises of an array of professionals who play different roles in the system. For instance, nurses are concerned with providing nursing care to patients, whereas physicians deal with the patients' treatment. As such, the US healthcare system involves many parties who work in collaboration to ensure that patients receive quality care for improved outcomes. Therefore, there is the need for developing reliable information system that will enhance communication between nurses and other stakeholders involved in the healthcare services delivery. It is regrettable that the current information infrastructure encompasses faults in many aspects. For instance, workforce data is not available, and this is considered as a significant drawback in workforce planning.

Recommendations

In ensuring a transient transformation of the US healthcare system under the ACA reforms, IOM offers 8 recommendations that will enhance the achievement of the desired targets.

Recommendation #1

Recommendation one aims at removing the scope of nursing practice barriers that seem to have hindered progress in the current healthcare system. They observe "advanced practice registered nurses should be able to practice to the full extent of their education and training" (p. 278). As such, it advices the congress and legislature to carry out the amendment of some legislation, in order to lift the existing barriers witnessed in the scope of the nursing practice. It requires the congress to carry out amendments on the Medicare program, in order to allow an extension of nursing care to patients in hospice and other advanced nursing facilities. It also requires the congress to extend the scope of nursing under the state law, more or less the same as it is the case for physicians.

On the other hand, IOM advises the state legislatures to reform the scope of nursing practice. As such, IOM (2010b) "requires third-party payers that participate in fee-for-service payment arrangements to provide direct reimbursement to advanced practice registered nurses who are practicing within their scope of practice under state law" (p. 1). It also advices the centers for Medicaid and Medicare services to extend eligibility to registered nurses.

Recommendation #2

The second recommendation deals with the expansion of opportunities for nurses. This is expected to enhance improvement efforts through collaboration. Expansion of opportunities to nurses includes their participation in research and other healthcare related investigations that are aimed at improving healthcare service delivery in the US healthcare system. As such, IOM requires the Center for Medicaid and Medicare to support the development of appropriate models of payment for registered nurses, in order to acknowledge leadership roles of the nursing professionals. This will help in reducing costs and improving health outcomes.

On the other hand, research models of care are supposed to be developed in addition to the incorporation of innovative solutions, in order to ensure the nurses' potential is utilized for the improvement of care in a care setting. However, this requires funding from the relevant organizations including private and public funders. In achieving this objective, IOM (2010b) states "Health care organizations should engage nurses and other front-line staff to work with developers and manufacturers in the design, development, purchase, implementation, and evaluation of medical and health devices and health information technology products" (p. 2).

Recommendation #3

The third recommendation calls for the implementation of nurse residency program that will help transitioning nurses to receive appropriate orientation in the healthcare system. Some of the bodies responsible for ensuring that pre-licensure or graduate nurses are absorbed into the healthcare system include state boards of nursing, healthcare organizations, the federal government and accrediting bodies. IOM recommends that these bodies to work in collaboration in designing efficient residency programs for new nurses entering the nursing profession. Therefore, these organizations are supposed to fund the establishment of such programs, in order to enhance the expansion of nurses' competencies and to improve the patients' outcomes (2010). In addition, this approach will promote the retention of nurses in the healthcare system; an aspect that has always presented enormous challenges to the US public healthcare system. It is reported that, retention of nurses in the US healthcare system has hindered the delivery of quality care to patients because the workforce is not adequate to meet the needs of the US population. In the recent years, nurses have been shifting to other areas of healthcare system that offer an appreciable compensation and friendly working environment (Aries, Middaugh & Nickitas, 2010).

Recommendation #4

The fourth recommendation seems to be related to the Millennium Development Goals (MDGs) because it seeks to increase the percentage of baccalaureate nurses to about 80 percent by 2020. Currently, workforce data indicates that there are about 50 percent of nurses with baccalaureate degrees. This proportion is relatively low because the healthcare demands of the US citizens are increasing day-by-day. Therefore, increasing the proportion of baccalaureate degree nurses is deemed necessary, in order to ensure that the US system is not burdened with patients' demand for nursing care. In theory, increasing the proportion of baccalaureate degree nurses from 50 to 80 percent is not an easy task. This is so because; there are many stakeholders involved in the nursing education who need to collaborate in ensuring the rate of enrollment into the nursing degree programs is improved. In overcoming this barrier, IOM recommends the collaboration of all academic nurse leaders across nursing schools in defining appropriate academic pathways for nursing students. In addition, this collaboration is expected to promote seamless access to higher levels of education for nurses.

Recommendation #5

On the other hand, IOM's fifth recommendation seeks to increase the number of doctorate nurses by half before the year 2020. They observe "schools of nursing, with support from private and public funders, academic administrators and university trustees, and accrediting bodies should double the number of nurses with a doctorate by 2020 to add to the cadre of nurse faculty and researchers" (p. 4). To achieve this target, IOM recommends that all accredited nursing schools ensure that at least ten percent of graduate nurses advance to a doctorate nursing program within five years of graduation with baccalaureate degrees. Therefore, National League for Nursing Accrediting Commission and the Commission on Collegiate Nursing Education are supposed to monitors the progress of all accredited nursing institutions to ensure this objective is met.

Consequently, funding for doctorate students should be made available for doctorate and master's nurse students. This will help enhancing the diversity of the nurse faculty. In addition, IOM recommends that university trustees and administrators should review salary and benefit packages to ensure that the recruitment and retention of highly qualified clinical and academic nursing faculty is created in a market competitive environment.

Recommendation #6

The sixth recommendation discusses the elements that will ensure that nurses engage in lifelong learning. That is why IOM (2010b) advises "Faculty should partner with health care organizations to develop and prioritize competencies so curricula can be updated regularly to ensure that graduates at all levels are prepared to meet the current and future health needs of the population" (p. 5).

It is also believed that a reliable transformation of nursing education requires that nurses possess high academic standards, in order to gain adequate professional skills. Ordinarily, nursing profession presents an array of challenges which require highly competent professionals to solve them. According to the IOM (2010a), "nursing education at all levels needs to provide a better understanding of and experience in care management, quality improvement methods, systems-level change management, and the reconceptualized roles of nurses in a reformed health care system" (p. 163). It is for this sense that an improved education system which will produce competent nursing professionals is required for healthcare transformation.

Recommendation #7

In the seventh recommendation, IOM seeks to ensure that nurses lead change in the advancement of the healthcare. In this regard, IOM (2010b) states "nurses should take responsibility for their personal and professional growth by continuing their education and seeking opportunities to develop and exercise their leadership skills" (p. 6). In the recent years, it has turned out that leadership in the nursing profession forms one of the most significant elements of the nursing practice. This is, probably why IOM (2010a) states "nurses have the opportunity to play a central role in transforming the health care system to create a more accessible, high-quality, and value-driven environment for patients" (p. 85).

Therefore, this report recommends "all nurses must be leaders in the design, implementation, and evaluation of, as well as advocacy for, the ongoing reforms to the system that will be needed" (p. 221). This will create a significant impact on personal qualities on nurses because it will foster leadership capability in all nurses. As a result, nurses will look more of leaders to the public than just care providers.

Recommendation #8

Finally, the 8th recommendation is concerned with building a reliable infrastructure for the collection and analysis of inter-professional healthcare workforce information. It is recommended that healthcare workforce requirements should be updated through the collection and analysis of the relevant data, in order to ensure improved access to healthcare information by the public and other concerned parties. Therefore, some regulatory bodies including the Health Resources and Services Administration and Government Accountability Office should provide oversight in this aspect which is to be carried out by the National Health Care Workforce Commission.

In attaining the expected objectives, IOM recommends for the increase of the sample size and the expansion of data collection, especially regarding advanced practice registered nurses. In addition, the Health Resources and Services Administration Office is required to ensure that fielding is done every other year, apart from releasing survey results with a short duration.

Conclusion

Conclusively, the 2010 IOM recommendations on transforming nursing practice, education and leadership appear to be consistent with the current US healthcare reforms. IOM (2010a) states

"Achieving transformation will require remodeling many aspects of the health care system; this is especially true for the nursing profession, the largest segment of the health care workforce" (p. 1). This is so because; the implementation of these recommendations will impact positively on the nursing education and profession; thus, achieving the desired goals of healthcare. IOM (2010a) states the principal goal as "care that is centered on [the patients'] unique needs" (p. 85).

It is apparent that the current IOM recommendations have an extensive impact on the nursing profession. For instance, IOM recommendations on nursing education will cause significant changes in educational perspectives of most nurses. This is so because; it recommends that nurses should pursue their education the advanced level to gain professional competence. As such, this recommendation puts nurses on lifelong learning, compulsorily. In addition, strict accreditation, licensing and certification of nursing students may present academic challenges to nursing students. However, it is worth noting that the implementation of IOM's recommendations will enhance professional competence among nurses.

References

Aries, N., Middaugh, D. J., & Nickitas, D. M. (2010). *Policy and Politics for Nurses and Other Health Professionals*. Burlington, MA: Jones & Bartlett Publishers.

IOM (2010a). *The Future of Nursing: Leading Change, Advancing Health*. Washington, D.C: The National Academies Press. Retrieved from http://www.nap.edu/catalog.php?record_id=12956

IOM (2010b). *The Future of Nursing Leading Change, Advancing Health Advising the Nation/Improving health: Report Recommendations*. Retrieved from http://www.iom.edu/~/media/Files/Report%20Files/2010/The-Future-of-Nursing/Future%20of%20Nursing%202010%20Recommendations.pdf

YOUR KNOWLEDGE HAS VALUE

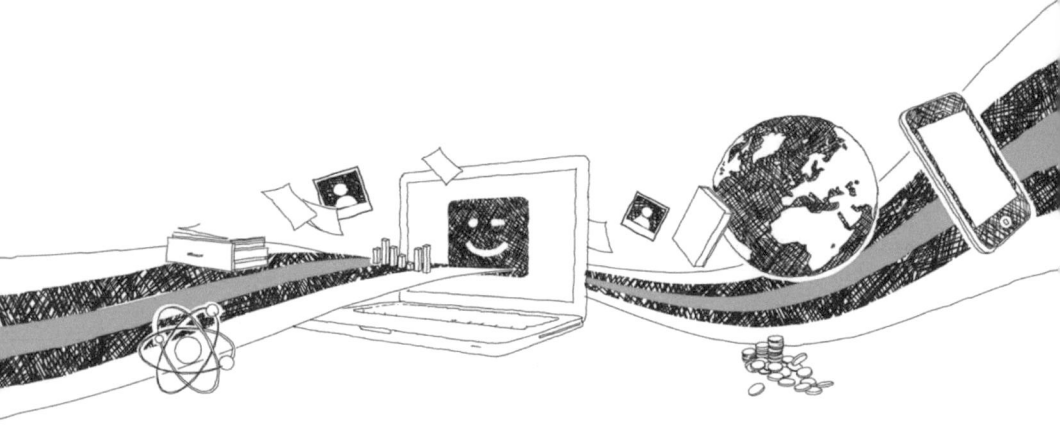

- We will publish your bachelor's and
  master's thesis, essays and papers

- Your own eBook and book -
  sold worldwide in all relevant shops

- Earn money with each sale

Upload your text at www.GRIN.com
and publish for free

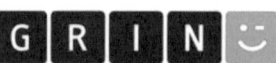